SMOOTHIES FOR TYPE 2 DIABETES

Nourish, Energize with Guilt Free Blood Sugar Friendly Smoothies and Juices

Kelly Walterhouse

@2024 Kelly Walterhouse

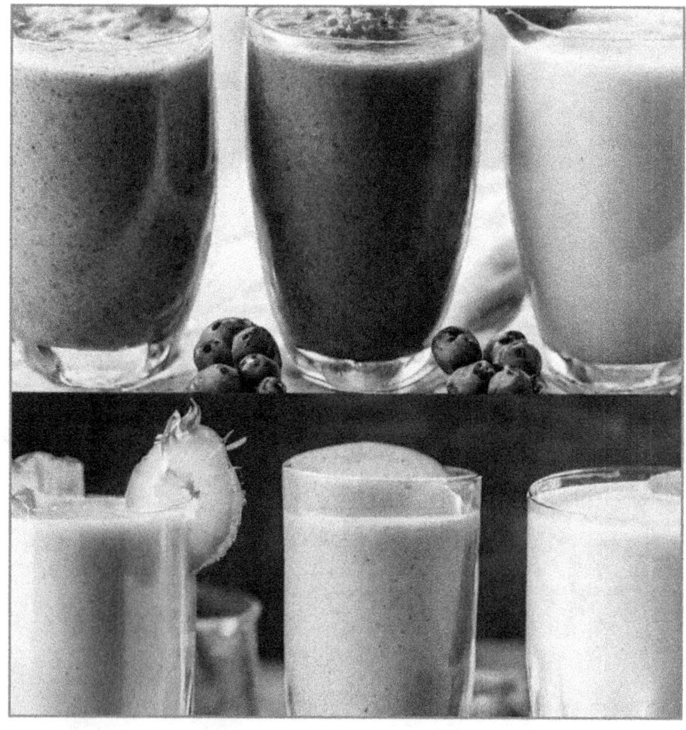

TABLE OF CONTENT

Introduction to Smoothies for Type 2 Diabetes: A Nutritional Approach

Understanding Type 2 Diabetes and Nutrition:

Type 2 diabetes is a metabolic disorder characterized by elevated blood sugar levels resulting from insulin resistance or insufficient insulin production. Nutrition plays a pivotal role in managing this condition, and individuals diagnosed with type 2 diabetes often seek dietary solutions to maintain blood sugar levels within a healthy range. It is crucial to comprehend the impact of different foods on blood sugar and adopt a wellbalanced approach to nutrition.

In the context of type 2 diabetes, carbohydrates directly influence blood glucose levels. The body breaks down carbohydrates into sugar, affecting blood sugar levels. Therefore, managing carbohydrate intake is a key aspect of diabetes management. It involves making mindful choices regarding the types of carbohydrates consumed, focusing on those with a lower glycemic index to minimize spikes in blood sugar.

The Importance of Smoothies in a Diabetic Diet:

Smoothies present a versatile and convenient option for individuals with type 2 diabetes to incorporate a variety of nutrientdense ingredients into their diet. When carefully crafted, smoothies can offer a balanced combination of carbohydrates, proteins, healthy fats, vitamins, and minerals. The liquid form of smoothies allows for easy digestion and absorption of essential nutrients, making them a practical choice for those with diabetes.

One of the significant advantages of smoothies is the potential to customize recipes based on individual dietary preferences and nutritional needs. This adaptability empowers individuals to create delicious and satisfying smoothies while adhering to the dietary guidelines recommended for managing type 2 diabetes.

By using whole, fresh ingredients, individuals can avoid added sugars, artificial sweeteners, and processed foods that may negatively impact blood sugar levels. Smoothies provide an opportunity to increase the intake of fruits, vegetables, and other fiberrich foods, which contribute to satiety and help regulate blood sugar.

Moreover, the combination of fiber and protein in smoothies can slow down the absorption of sugar, preventing rapid spikes in blood glucose levels. This is particularly important for individuals with diabetes, as stable blood sugar levels contribute to overall health and wellbeing.

Creating a diabeticfriendly smoothie involves selecting ingredients with a low glycemic index, such as leafy greens, berries, and nuts. Additionally, incorporating sources of healthy fats, such as avocados or chia seeds, can enhance the nutritional profile and contribute to a sense of fullness.

As individuals with type 2 diabetes often need to monitor their weight, smoothies can be a valuable tool in achieving and maintaining a healthy weight. The controlled portions and nutrient density of smoothies make them an effective option for those looking to manage their caloric intake while ensuring they receive essential nutrients.

In summary, the introduction to smoothies for type 2 diabetes emphasizes the importance of understanding the relationship between nutrition and diabetes management. Smoothies offer a practical and enjoyable way for individuals to embrace a healthful diet, contributing to overall wellbeing and improved blood sugar control. The following sections will delve into specific categories of smoothies designed to cater to the diverse tastes and nutritional needs of individuals with type 2 diabetes.

2. Basics of Diabetic Friendly Smoothies

Creating diabetic friendly smoothies involves a thoughtful combination of ingredients, mindful portion control, and vigilant monitoring of sugar content. For individuals managing diabetes, adopting a balanced and nutritious diet is crucial, and incorporating smoothies can be a delicious and convenient way to achieve this.

Choosing the Right Ingredients

The foundation of a diabetic friendly smoothie lies in selecting ingredients that not only satisfy taste buds but also contribute to stable blood sugar levels. Opting for whole, unprocessed foods is a fundamental principle. Fresh fruits, vegetables, and sources of lean protein are excellent starting points.

1. **Fruits:** While fruits contain natural sugars, choosing those with a lower glycemic index is advisable. Berries, such as blueberries, strawberries, and raspberries, are rich in antioxidants and relatively

low in sugar. Avocado is another excellent addition, offering healthy fats that help slow down the absorption of sugars.

2. Vegetables: Incorporating leafy greens like spinach and kale adds essential vitamins and minerals without significantly impacting blood sugar levels. These vegetables are also low in carbohydrates, making them a smart choice for diabeticfriendly smoothies.

3. Protein: Including a source of protein is vital for satiety and blood sugar control. Opt for options like Greek yogurt, unsweetened almond milk, or protein powder without added sugars. Protein not only helps stabilize blood sugar but also provides a feeling of fullness, reducing the temptation to snack on less healthy options.

4. Healthy Fats: Adding sources of healthy fats, such as nuts, seeds, or a spoonful of nut butter, contributes to a smoother texture and helps slow down the digestion of carbohydrates, preventing rapid spikes in blood sugar.

5. Liquid Base: Carefully choosing the liquid base is essential. Unsweetened almond milk, coconut water, or plain water are preferable to highsugar fruit juices or sweetened yogurts. These options provide hydration without adding excessive sugar to the smoothie.

Portion Control and Monitoring Sugar Content

1. Mindful Portions: While nutrient dense, even diabeticfriendly ingredients can contribute to an excess of calories and carbohydrates if not consumed in moderation. Controlling portion sizes is key to managing blood sugar levels. Consider using measuring cups or a kitchen scale to ensure accuracy in ingredient quantities.

2. Limiting HighGlycemic Ingredients: Some fruits, even though nutritious, can be higher in natural sugars. Moderation is crucial when incorporating them into smoothies. For example, bananas and mangoes, while delicious, should be used sparingly to prevent sudden spikes in blood sugar.

3. Monitoring Added Sugars: Be cautious of hidden sugars in ingredients like flavored yogurt, sweetened nut milks, or prepackaged protein powders. Reading nutrition labels is essential to identify and avoid added sugars that can compromise the diabeticfriendly nature of the smoothie.

4. Balancing Macronutrients: Achieving a balance of macronutrients – carbohydrates, proteins, and fats – in the smoothie is essential for stable blood sugar levels. Striking the right balance helps prevent rapid increases or decreases in blood glucose, promoting a sustained release of energy.

5. Regular Blood Sugar Monitoring: Individuals with diabetes should regularly monitor their blood sugar levels, especially after consuming a smoothie or any meal. This practice allows for adjustments in diet and medication if needed, ensuring optimal blood sugar control.

In conclusion, crafting diabetic friendly smoothies involves a thoughtful selection of ingredients, mindful portion control, and vigilant monitoring of sugar content. By incorporating nutrientdense and lowglycemic ingredients, paying attention to portion sizes, and being aware of hidden sugars, individuals with diabetes can enjoy delicious and healthful smoothies as part of their balanced diet. Always consult with a healthcare professional or nutritionist to tailor smoothie recipes to specific dietary needs and health goals.

3. Nutrient Rich Green Smoothies

Green Powerhouse

Ingredients:

- 1 cup spinach
- 1/2 cucumber
- 1/2 avocado
- 1/2 lemon (juiced)
- 1 cup unsweetened almond milk

Instructions:

Blend all ingredients until smooth.

Benefits: Packed with fiber, healthy fats, and vitamins, this smoothie aids in maintaining steady blood sugar levels.

Berry Green Fusion

Ingredients:

- 1 cup kale
- 1/2 cup blueberries
- 1 tablespoon chia seeds
- 1 cup water or green tea

Instructions:

Blend all ingredients until well combined.

Benefits: Rich in antioxidants and fiber, this smoothie supports heart health and helps regulate blood sugar.

Cucumber Spinach Delight

Ingredients:

- 1 cup spinach
- 1/2 cucumber
- 1/2 green apple
- 1 tablespoon flaxseeds
- 1 cup water

Instructions:

Blend until smooth.

Benefits: Low in sugar, high in fiber, and hydrating, this smoothie contributes to a diabetesfriendly diet.

Avocado Mint Magic

Ingredients:

- 1 cup kale
- 1/2 avocado
- 1/4 cup fresh mint leaves
- 1/2 lime (juiced)
- 1 cup coconut water

Instructions:

Blend until creamy.

Benefits: Provides healthy fats, vitamins, and minerals, aiding in blood sugar control and overall wellbeing.

Ginger Green Goodness

Ingredients:

- 1 cup spinach
- 1/2 inch fresh ginger (peeled)
- 1/2 green pear
- 1 tablespoon hemp seeds
- 1 cup water

Instructions:

Blend until smooth.

Benefits: Ginger may help lower blood sugar levels, and combined with fiberrich greens, this smoothie is a diabetesfriendly option.

Pineapple Kale Twist

Ingredients:

- 1 cup kale
- 1/2 cup pineapple (fresh or frozen)
- 1/2 cucumber
- 1/2 lemon (juiced)

- 1 cup water

Instructions:

Blend until well combined.

Benefits: Low in sugar and rich in vitamin C, this smoothie supports immune health and regulates blood sugar.

Coconut Spinach Surprise

Ingredients:

- 1 cup spinach
- 1/2 cup coconut milk (unsweetened)
- 1/2 cup zucchini
- 1 tablespoon chia seeds
- 1/2 teaspoon cinnamon

Instructions:

Blend until creamy.

Benefits: Provides a creamy texture with healthy fats and added fiber, supporting blood sugar management.

Broccoli Blueberry Boost

Ingredients:

- 1 cup broccoli florets
- 1/2 cup blueberries
- 1/2 banana (optional)
- 1 tablespoon almond butter
- 1 cup water or almond milk

Instructions:

Blend until smooth.

Benefits: Broccoli adds fiber and nutrients, while blueberries contribute antioxidants, creating a diabetesfriendly combination.

Mango Spinach Sensation

Ingredients:

- 1 cup spinach
- 1/2 cup mango (fresh or frozen)
- 1/2 cucumber
- 1 tablespoon flaxseeds
- 1 cup coconut water

Instructions:

Blend until well combined.

Benefits: Mango adds natural sweetness, and the combination of ingredients offers a refreshing and nutritious choice for those with diabetes.

Turmeric Green Elixir

Ingredients:

- 1 cup kale
- 1/2 teaspoon turmeric powder
- 1/2 avocado
- 1/2 lime (juiced)
- 1 cup green tea

Instructions:

Blend until creamy.

Benefits: Turmeric may have antiinflammatory properties, and when combined with nutrientrich greens, this smoothie can be beneficial for managing inflammation associated with diabetes.

4. Berrylicious Smoothies

Berry Protein Powerhouse

Ingredients:

- 1 cup mixed berries (strawberries, blueberries, raspberries)
- 1/2 cup Greek yogurt (unsweetened)
- 1 scoop unflavored protein powder
- 1 tablespoon chia seeds
- 1 cup unsweetened almond milk

Instructions:

Blend berries, Greek yogurt, protein powder, and chia seeds until smooth. Add almond milk gradually and blend until desired consistency.

Benefits: This smoothie is rich in protein, fiber, and antioxidants, supporting blood sugar control.

Strawberry Avocado Elixir

Ingredients:

- 1 cup strawberries (fresh or frozen)
- 1/2 ripe avocado
- 1 tablespoon flaxseeds
- 1 cup spinach leaves
- 1/2 cup water

Instructions:

Blend strawberries, avocado, flaxseeds, and spinach until creamy. Add water gradually for the desired thickness.

Benefits: Avocado contributes healthy fats, promoting satiety and stable blood sugar levels.

Blueberry Almond Bliss

Ingredients:

- 1 cup blueberries (fresh or frozen)
- 1/4 cup almonds (unsalted)
- 1/2 cup plain Greek yogurt
- 1 tablespoon almond butter

- 1 cup unsweetened almond milk

Instructions:

Blend blueberries, almonds, Greek yogurt, and almond butter until smooth. Add almond milk gradually for desired consistency.

Benefits: Almonds add protein and healthy fats, making this smoothie diabetesfriendly.

Raspberry Green Delight

Ingredients:

- 1/2 cup raspberries (fresh or frozen)
- 1 cup kale leaves (stems removed)
- 1/2 cucumber (peeled)
- 1 tablespoon hemp seeds
- 1 cup coconut water

Instructions:

Blend raspberries, kale, cucumber, and hemp seeds until well combined. Add coconut water gradually until desired thickness.

Benefits: Low in sugar, this smoothie offers a nutrient boost with greens and berries.

Mixed Berry Citrus Splash

Ingredients:

- 1/2 cup mixed berries (strawberries, blueberries, blackberries)
- 1/2 orange (peeled)
- 1 tablespoon flaxseeds
- 1 cup water or green tea (unsweetened)

Instructions:

Blend mixed berries, orange, and flaxseeds until smooth. Add water or green tea gradually to reach the desired consistency.

Benefits: The addition of citrus provides a refreshing twist with added fiber.

Blackberry Walnut Wonder

Ingredients:

- 1 cup blackberries (fresh or frozen)
- 1/4 cup walnuts
- 1/2 cup plain Greek yogurt
- 1 tablespoon chia seeds
- 1 cup unsweetened almond milk

Instructions:

Blend blackberries, walnuts, Greek yogurt, and chia seeds until creamy. Gradually add almond milk for desired thickness.

Benefits: Walnuts contribute omega3 fatty acids, promoting heart health.

Mango Raspberry Medley

Ingredients:

- 1/2 cup raspberries (fresh or frozen)
- 1/2 cup mango chunks
- 1/2 cup plain Greek yogurt
- 1 tablespoon pumpkin seeds
- 1 cup water or coconut water (unsweetened)

Instructions:

Blend raspberries, mango, Greek yogurt, and pumpkin seeds until smooth. Add water or coconut water gradually for desired consistency.

Benefits: This smoothie combines the sweetness of mango with the tartness of raspberries.

Cherry Almond Delight

Ingredients:

- 1 cup cherries (pitted, fresh or frozen)
- 1/4 cup almonds (unsalted)
- 1/2 cup plain Greek yogurt
- 1 tablespoon flaxseeds
- 1 cup unsweetened almond milk

Instructions:

Blend cherries, almonds, Greek yogurt, and flaxseeds until creamy. Gradually add almond milk for the desired thickness.

Benefits:. Cherries provide antioxidants and are lower in sugar compared to some other fruits.

Pomegranate Berry Burst

Ingredients:

- 1/2 cup mixed berries (strawberries, blueberries, blackberries)
- 1/2 cup pomegranate seeds
- 1/2 cup plain Greek yogurt
- 1 tablespoon chia seeds
- 1 cup water or green tea (unsweetened)

Instructions:

Blend mixed berries, pomegranate seeds, Greek yogurt, and chia seeds until smooth. Add water or green tea gradually for desired consistency.

Benefits: Pomegranate seeds add a burst of flavor and antioxidants to this smoothie.

Cranberry Cinnamon Spice

Ingredients:

- 1/2 cup cranberries (fresh or unsweetened dried)
- 1/2 banana
- 1/2 teaspoon cinnamon
- 1/2 cup plain Greek yogurt
- 1 cup water or almond milk (unsweetened)

Instructions:

Blend cranberries, banana, cinnamon, and Greek yogurt until smooth. Add water or almond milk gradually for the desired consistency.

Benefits: Cinnamon adds flavor without additional sugar, making this a diabetesfriendly choice.

5. Citrus Infusions

Citrus Basil Delight

Ingredients:

- 1 orange, sliced
- 1 lemon, sliced
- Fresh basil leaves

Instructions:

Combine orange and lemon slices in a pitcher. Add fresh basil leaves. Fill the pitcher with water and refrigerate for a few hours.

Benefits: Basil adds flavor without extra sugar, and citrus fruits provide vitamins and antioxidants.

Lime and Mint Zest

Ingredients:

- 2 limes, sliced
- Fresh mint leaves

Instructions:

Place lime slices in a pitcher. Add fresh mint leaves. Fill the pitcher with water and let it chill in the refrigerator.

Benefits: Mint aids digestion, and limes offer a burst of vitamin C without spiking blood sugar.

Grapefruit Rosemary Infusion:

Ingredients:

- 1 grapefruit, sliced
- Fresh rosemary sprigs

Instructions:

Combine grapefruit slices and rosemary in a pitcher.Add water and refrigerate for a citrusy boost.

Benefits: Grapefruit supports weight management and rosemary adds a unique flavor.

Orange and Ginger Elixir

Ingredients:

- 2 oranges, sliced
- Fresh ginger slices

Instructions:

Place orange slices and ginger in a pitcher. Add water and refrigerate to let the flavors meld.

Benefits: Ginger may help lower blood sugar levels, and oranges provide natural sweetness.

Mandarin Mint Fusion:

Ingredients:

- 1 cup mandarin segments
- Fresh mint leaves

Instructions:

1. Mix mandarin segments and mint in a pitcher.

Add water and refrigerate for a refreshing infusion.

Benefits: Mandarins are low in sugar, and mint adds a pleasant aroma.

Lemon Thyme Serenity

Ingredients:

- 2 lemons, sliced
- Fresh thyme sprigs

Instructions:

Combine lemon slices and thyme in a pitcher. Fill the pitcher with water and chill for a soothing beverage.

Benefits: Thyme adds a unique herbal note, and lemons provide a burst of vitamin C.

Tangerine and Cinnamon Spice

Ingredients:

- 2 tangerines, sliced
- Cinnamon sticks

Instructions:

Place tangerine slices and cinnamon sticks in a pitcher. Add water and let it infuse for a subtle spiced flavor.

Benefits: Cinnamon may help improve insulin sensitivity.

Pomelo Mint Cooler

Ingredients:

- pomelo, segmented
- Fresh mint leaves

Instructions:

Mix pomelo segments and mint in a pitcher. . Fill the pitcher with water and refrigerate for a tropical twist.

Benefits: Pomelo is a lowsugar citrus option, and mint aids digestion.

Lemon and Blueberry Bliss:

Ingredients:

- 1 lemon, sliced
- 1/2 cup blueberries

Instructions:

Combine lemon slices and blueberries in a pitcher. Add water and refrigerate for a refreshing and antioxidantrich infusion.

Benefits: Blueberries are low in sugar and high in antioxidants.

Citrus Splash with Rose Petals:

Ingredients:

- Mix of citrus slices (orange, lemon, lime)
- Fresh rose petals (edible, pesticidefree)

Instructions:

. Combine citrus slices and rose petals in a pitcher.

Add water and refrigerate for a visually appealing and fragrant infusion.

Benefits: Citrus provides vitamins, while rose petals add a delicate flavor without added sugars.

6. Protein Packed Options

Berry Protein Blast

Ingredients:

- 1/2 cup mixed berries (blueberries, strawberries, raspberries)
- 1/2 cup Greek yogurt (unsweetened)
- 1 scoop protein powder (whey or plantbased)
- 1 tablespoon chia seeds
- 1 cup unsweetened almond milk

Instructions:

Blend all ingredients until smooth. Pour into a glass and enjoy.

Benefits Berries are rich in antioxidants and fiber.

Greek yogurt provides protein without added sugars. Chia seeds add omega3 fatty acids for heart health.

Green Power Protein

Ingredients:

- 1 cup spinach
- 1/2 banana (preferably greentipped)
- 1/2 cup cucumber
- 1 scoop protein powder (unflavored)
- 1 tablespoon almond butter
- 1 cup water or unsweetened almond milk

Instructions:

Blend all ingredients until creamy. . Pour into a glass and enjoy.

Benefits Lowglycemic index ingredients.

Spinach and cucumber provide essential nutrients.

Avocado Berry Bliss

Ingredients:

- 1/2 avocado
- 1/2 cup mixed berries
- 1 scoop protein powder (vanilla or unflavored)
- 1 tablespoon flaxseeds
- 1 cup unsweetened coconut water

Instructions:

Blend all ingredients until smooth. Pour into a glass and savor.

Benefits Avocado contributes healthy fats.

Flaxseeds add fiber for better blood sugar control.

Peanut Butter Banana Protein

Ingredients:

- 1 banana
- 2 tablespoons peanut butter (unsweetened)
- 1 scoop protein powder (chocolate or unflavored)
- 1/2 cup plain Greek yogurt

- 1 cup unsweetened almond milk

Instructions:

Blend all ingredients until creamy. Pour into a glass and relish.

Benefits: Peanut butter provides protein and healthy fats. Banana adds natural sweetness and potassium.

. ChiaBerry Protein Delight

Ingredients:

- 1/4 cup chia seeds
- 1/2 cup mixed berries
- 1 scoop protein powder (unflavored)
- 1 tablespoon almond butter
- 1 cup unsweetened almond milk

Instructions:

Blend all ingredients except chia seeds until smooth Stir in chia seeds and let it sit for 10 minutes. . Pour into a glass and enjoy.

Benefits Chia seeds provide fiber and omega3 fatty acids. Berries contribute antioxidants.

Cocoa Almond Protein Shake

Ingredients:

- 1 scoop chocolate protein powder
- 1 tablespoon almond butter
- 1 tablespoon cocoa powder (unsweetened)
- 1/2 banana
- 1 cup unsweetened almond milk

Instructions:

Blend all ingredients until velvety. Pour into a glass and relish the chocolatey goodness.

Benefits: Cocoa powder adds a rich flavor without added sugars. Almond butter provides healthy fats.

Vanilla Cinnamon Protein Elixir

Ingredients:

- 1 scoop vanilla protein powder
- 1/2 teaspoon cinnamon
- 1/2 cup cottage cheese (lowfat)
- 1/2 cup unsweetened almond milk
- Ice cubes (optional)

Instructions:

Blend all ingredients until creamy. Add ice cubes if desired and blend again.   Pour into a glass and relish the vanillacinnamon blend.

Benefits Cinnamon may help improve insulin sensitivity. Cottage cheese adds protein and creaminess.

Mango Protein Paradise

Ingredients:

- 1/2 cup mango (frozen or fresh)
- 1 scoop protein powder (vanilla or unflavored)
- 1/2 cup plain Greek yogurt
- 1 tablespoon hemp seeds
- 1 cup water or coconut water

Instructions:

Blend all ingredients until smooth. Pour into a glass and enjoy the tropical goodness.

Benefits Mango adds natural sweetness with moderate impact on blood sugar. Hemp seeds provide omega3 fatty acids.

Coconut Berry Protein Fusion

Ingredients:

- 1/2 cup mixed berries
- 1 scoop protein powder (coconutflavored or unflavored)
- 1/4 cup coconut milk (unsweetened)
- 1/2 cup plain Greek yogurt
- 1/2 teaspoon coconut flakes (optional)

Instructions:

Blend all ingredients until creamy. Garnish with coconut flakes if desired. Pour into a glass and savor the tropical blend.

Benefits Coconut milk adds flavor without excessive sugar. Berries contribute antioxidants and fiber.

Almond Joy Protein Shake

Ingredients:

- 1 scoop chocolate protein powder

- 1 tablespoon almond butter

- 1/4 cup shredded coconut (unsweetened)

- 1/2 teaspoon almond extract

- 1 cup unsweetened almond milk

Instructions:

. Blend all ingredients until smooth. Pour into a glass and enjoy the almond joy flavor.

Benefits   Almond extract provides flavor without added sugars. Shredded coconut adds texture and healthy fats.

7. Low-Glycemic Fruit Smoothies

Berry Citrus Splash

Ingredients:

- 1/2 cup blueberries
- 1/2 cup raspberries
- 1/2 cup strawberries (sliced)
- 1/2 orange (peeled)
- 1 cup unsweetened almond milk

Instructions:

Combine all ingredients in a blender. Blend until smooth. Pour into a glass and enjoy!

Benefits Berries have a low glycemic index and are rich in antioxidants. Citrus fruits add a refreshing flavor without causing rapid blood sugar spikes.

Green Apple Cinnamon Delight

Ingredients:

- 1 green apple (cored and sliced)
- 1/2 teaspoon cinnamon
- 1 cup spinach leaves
- 1/2 avocado
- 1 cup water

Instructions:

Blend all ingredients until creamy. Adjust thickness with water as needed. . Pour into a glass and sprinkle a pinch of cinnamon on top.

Benefits Green apple and spinach are lowglycemic choices.Cinnamon may help improve insulin sensitivity.

Peach Almond Bliss

Ingredients:

- 1 cup sliced peaches (fresh or frozen)
- 1 tablespoon almond butter
- 1/2 cup Greek yogurt (unsweetened)
- 1/2 teaspoon vanilla extract
- 1 cup ice cubes

Instructions:

Blend all ingredients until smooth. Add more ice if a thicker consistency is desired. Pour into a glass and enjoy.

Benefits Peaches are a lowglycemic fruit. Almond butter provides healthy fats and protein for sustained energy.

Berry Spinach Powerhouse

Ingredients:

- 1/2 cup mixed berries (blueberries, strawberries, raspberries)
- 1 cup fresh spinach leaves
- 1/2 cup cucumber (sliced)
- 1/2 lemon (juiced)
- 1 cup water

Instructions:

Blend all ingredients until well combined. Adjust consistency with water if needed. Pour into a glass and garnish with a lemon slice.

Benefits Berries and spinach are low in sugar and high in fiber. Cucumber adds hydration without extra sugars.

Chia Berry Fusion

Ingredients:

- 1/2 cup mixed berries (strawberries, blackberries, raspberries)
- 1 tablespoon chia seeds
- 1/2 cup unsweetened coconut milk
- 1/2 cup Greek yogurt (unsweetened)
- 1/2 teaspoon honey (optional)

Instructions:

Blend berries, chia seeds, and coconut milk until smooth. Layer with Greek yogurt. Drizzle honey on top if desired.

Benefits Chia seeds provide fiber for blood sugar control. Greek yogurt offers protein for a balanced smoothie.

Avocado Mango Tango

Ingredients:

- 1/2 avocado
- 1/2 cup mango chunks (fresh or frozen)
- 1/2 cup spinach leaves
- 1/2 lime (juiced)
- 1 cup water

Instructions:

Blend all ingredients until creamy. Adjust consistency with water if needed. Pour into a glass and enjoy the tropical flavors.

Benefits Avocado and mango offer healthy fats and vitamins. Spinach adds fiber and essential nutrients.

Cranberry Orange Zest

Ingredients:

- 1/2 cup cranberries (fresh or unsweetened frozen)
- 1 orange (peeled)
- 1/2 cup Greek yogurt (unsweetened)
- 1/2 teaspoon grated ginger
- 1 cup ice cubes

Instructions:

Blend cranberries, orange, yogurt, and ginger until smooth. Add ice cubes for a refreshing texture. Pour into a glass and garnish with an orange zest.

Benefits Cranberries are low in sugar and may support urinary tract health. Ginger can have antiinflammatory effects.

Pineapple Mint Cooler

Ingredients:

- 1 cup pineapple chunks
- 1/2 cup cucumber (sliced)
- 1/4 cup fresh mint leaves
- 1/2 lime (juiced)
- 1 cup coconut water

Instructions:

Blend pineapple, cucumber, mint, lime juice, and coconut water. . Adjust sweetness with more pineapple if needed. Pour into a glass and enjoy the tropical freshness.

Benefits Pineapple adds natural sweetness with a relatively low glycemic index. Mint provides a refreshing taste without added sugars.

Strawberry Basil Breeze

Ingredients:

- 1 cup strawberries (hulled)
- 1/4 cup fresh basil leaves
- 1/2 cup Greek yogurt (unsweetened)
- 1/2 teaspoon honey (optional)
- 1 cup water

Instructions:

Blend strawberries, basil, yogurt, and honey until smooth. Adjust consistency with water as desired.. Pour into a glass and garnish with a basil leaf.

Benefits Strawberries are low in sugar and high in antioxidants. Basil adds a unique flavor while offering potential antiinflammatory properties.

Melon Mint Medley

Ingredients:

- 1 cup mixed melon cubes (cantaloupe, honeydew)
- 1/4 cup fresh mint leaves
- 1/2 cucumber (sliced)
- 1/2 lemon (juiced)
- 1 cup water

Instructions:

Blend melon, mint, cucumber, and lemon juice until well combined. Adjust thickness with water if needed. Pour into a glass and garnish with a mint sprig.

Benefits . Mint provides a refreshing taste without added sugars.

8. Hydration and Detox Smoothies

Berry Citrus Splash

Ingredients:

- 1 cup mixed berries (blueberries, strawberries, raspberries)
- 1/2 orange, peeled
- 1 cup spinach
- 1 cup water or coconut water

Instructions:

Blend all ingredients until smooth. This hydrating smoothie is rich in antioxidants and fiber, supporting blood sugar control.

Benefits: Berries are low in sugar and high in fiber, aiding in glucose regulation. Spinach provides essential vitamins and minerals.

Ingredients:

- 1 green apple, cored and chopped
- 1/2 cucumber, peeled
- Handful of mint leaves
- 1 cup water

Instructions:

Blend ingredients until well combined. This refreshing smoothie aids digestion and provides hydration without excess sugar.

Benefits: Green apples are low in sugar and high in fiber. Cucumber adds hydration, while mint supports digestion.

Cinnamon Spice Refresher

Ingredients:

- 1/2 banana
- 1/2 teaspoon cinnamon
- 1 tablespoon chia seeds
- 1 cup unsweetened almond milk

Instructions:

Blend until smooth. Cinnamon may help improve insulin sensitivity, making it suitable for a type 2 diabetes diet.

Benefits: Cinnamon may help regulate blood sugar levels, and chia seeds provide omega3 fatty acids and fiber.

Pineapple Ginger Zing

Ingredients:

- 1 cup fresh pineapple chunks
- 1 teaspoon grated ginger
- 1 cup kale leaves
- 1 cup coconut water

Instructions:

Blend ingredients until smooth. Pineapple adds natural sweetness, while ginger aids digestion.

Benefits: Pineapple contains bromelain, known for antiinflammatory properties, and kale is low in carbs and high in nutrients.

Citrus Mint Cooler

Ingredients:

- 1/2 grapefruit, peeled
- 1/2 lemon, peeled
- Handful of fresh mint leaves
- 1 cup water

Instructions:

Blend until smooth. This citrusy smoothie is hydrating and low in sugar.

Benefits: Citrus fruits are low in sugar, and mint supports digestion. The high water content aids in hydration.

Turmeric Mango Delight:

Ingredients:

- 1/2 cup mango chunks
- 1/2 teaspoon turmeric powder
- 1 tablespoon flaxseeds
- 1 cup water or unsweetened coconut milk

Instructions:

Blend until creamy. Turmeric provides antiinflammatory benefits.

Benefits: Turmeric has antiinflammatory properties, and flaxseeds offer fiber and healthy fats.

Berry Beet Boost:

Ingredients:

- 1/2 cup mixed berries
- 1/2 small beet, peeled and chopped
- 1 tablespoon hemp seeds
- 1 cup water or green tea (cooled)

Instructions:

Blend until well combined. Beets provide nutrients without spiking blood sugar.

Benefits: Berries are low in sugar, and beets offer essential vitamins and minerals. Hemp seeds add protein and omega3 fatty acids.

Avocado Cucumber Lime Elixir

Ingredients:

- 1/2 avocado
- 1/2 cucumber, peeled
- Juice of 1 lime
- 1 cup water or coconut water

Instructions:

Blend until smooth. Avocado provides healthy fats for sustained energy.

Benefits: Avocado adds healthy fats, while cucumber and lime contribute to hydration without excessive sugars.

Ginger Peach Bliss:

Ingredients:

- 1/2 cup peach slices (fresh or frozen)
- 1 teaspoon grated ginger
- 1 tablespoon chia seeds
- 1 cup unsweetened almond milk

Instructions:

Blend until creamy. Ginger aids digestion and adds a zesty flavor.

Benefits: Peaches are lower in sugar, and ginger supports digestion and has antiinflammatory properties.

Spinach Pineapple Protein Refuel:

Ingredients:

- Handful of spinach
- 1 cup fresh pineapple chunks
- 1 scoop protein powder (unsweetened)
- 1 cup water or unsweetened almond milk

Instructions:

Blend until smooth. This smoothie offers protein for satiety and nutrients from spinach and pineapple.

Benefits: Spinach is nutrientdense, and pineapple adds natural sweetness. Protein powder supports muscle health and helps control hunger.

9. Dessert Inspired Treats

CocoaBerry Delight:

Ingredients:

- 1/2 cup mixed berries (blueberries, raspberries)
- 1 tablespoon unsweetened cocoa powder
- 1 cup unsweetened almond milk
- Ice cubes (optional)

Instructions:

Blend for a guilt free chocolatey treat.

Benefits The antioxidants in berries and minimal sugar content support diabetes management. Berries also offer fiber, promoting steady blood sugar levels.

Vanilla Almond Dream:

Ingredients:

- 1/2 teaspoon vanilla extract
- 1 tablespoon almond butter
- 1/2 banana
- 1 cup unsweetened coconut milk

Instructions:

Blend for a creamy dessertlike flavor.

Benefits Healthy fats from almond butter contribute to stable blood sugar levels. The banana adds natural sweetness without spiking blood glucose.

Cinnamon Roll Bliss

Ingredients:

- 1/2 apple, cored and chopped
- 1/2 teaspoon ground cinnamon
- 1 cup spinach
- 1 cup unsweetened almond milk

Instructions:

Blend for a tasty cinnamon roll flavor.

Benefits The fiber in apple and spinach supports blood sugar control. Cinnamon may enhance insulin sensitivity.

= Peanut Butter Banana Swirl

Ingredients:

- 1/2 banana
- 1 tablespoon natural peanut butter
- 1 cup unsweetened soy milk
- Ice cubes (optional)

Instructions:

Blend for a delightful, diabetesfriendly dessert.

Benefits The protein in peanut butter and natural sweetness of banana make it satisfying. The combination provides a good balance of protein and healthy fats.

Mango Lassi Delight:

Ingredients:

- 1/2 cup fresh mango chunks
- 1/2 cup Greek yogurt (unsweetened)
- 1/2 teaspoon cardamom
- 1 cup water

Instructions:

Blend for a taste of the classic Indian dessert.

Benefits Probiotics from Greek yogurt add a healthful touch. Mango, in moderation, provides natural sweetness with a lower glycemic index.

Berries and Cream Fantasy

Ingredients:

- 1/2 cup mixed berries (strawberries, blueberries)
- 1/4 cup cottage cheese (lowfat)
- 1 teaspoon vanilla extract
- 1 cup unsweetened almond milk

Instructions:

Blend for a creamy, proteinrich treat.

Benefits Cottage cheese provides a satisfying texture. The protein and healthy fats help with satiety and blood sugar control.

Chia Chocolate Pudding Shake

Ingredients:

- 1 tablespoon chia seeds
- 1 tablespoon unsweetened cocoa powder
- 1/2 teaspoon vanilla extract
- 1 cup unsweetened coconut milk

Instructions:

Blend for a healthy chocolate treat

Benefits. Chia seeds add fiber and a puddinglike consistency. The fiber content aids in slowing down sugar absorption.

Apple Pie Smoothie:

Ingredients:

- 1/2 apple, cored and chopped
- 1/2 teaspoon ground cinnamon
- 1 tablespoon oats (rolled or steelcut)
- 1 cup unsweetened almond milk

Instructions:

Blend for an apple pieinspired delight.

Benefits The oats contribute fiber for blood sugar stability. The combination offers a dessertlike flavor with controlled sugar content.

Pumpkin Spice Elegance:

Ingredients:

- 1/2 cup pumpkin puree (unsweetened)
- 1/2 teaspoon pumpkin spice blend
- 1 tablespoon flaxseeds (ground)
- 1 cup unsweetened almond milk

Instructions:

Blend for a festive treat.

Benefits Pumpkin is low in sugar, and flaxseeds add omega3 fatty acids. The fiber from pumpkin and flaxseeds supports blood sugar management.

Strawberry Cheesecake Indulgence:

Ingredients:

- 1/2 cup strawberries
- 1/4 cup cream cheese (lowfat)
- 1 teaspoon lemon juice
- 1 cup unsweetened almond milk

Instructions:

Blend for a cheesecake inspired treat

Benefits The combination provides a satisfying taste with controlled sugar content. The moderate use of cream cheese adds flavor without significantly impacting blood sugar levels.

10. Special Occasion Smoothies

Holiday Spice Surprise:

Ingredients:

- 1/2 apple, cored and chopped
- 1/2 teaspoon cinnamon
- Pinch of nutmeg
- 1 tablespoon chia seeds
- 1 cup unsweetened almond milk

Instructions:

Blend until the spices are well incorporated.

Benefits This smoothie brings warm holiday flavors with the added benefit of chia seeds for fiber and omega3 fatty acids.

Birthday Cake Celebration:

Ingredients:

- 1/2 banana
- 1 tablespoon almond butter
- 1/2 teaspoon vanilla extract
- 1 cup unsweetened coconut milk

Instructions:

Blend until creamy.

Benefits This smoothie offers the delightful taste of birthday cake with healthy fats and minimal sugar, making it a guiltfree celebration treat.

Tropical Paradise Splash:

Ingredients:

- 1/2 cup pineapple chunks
- 1/2 mango, peeled and chopped
- 1/2 cup coconut water
- Handful of spinach leaves

Instructions:

Blend until tropical bliss is achieved.

Benefits This smoothie combines the sweetness of tropical fruits with the nutritional boost of spinach, creating a refreshing celebration drink.

Cherry Blossom Celebration:

Ingredients:

- 1/2 cup cherries, pitted
- 1/2 cup strawberries
- 1/2 teaspoon almond extract
- 1 cup unsweetened almond milk

Instructions:

Blend until smooth.

Benefits Cherries and strawberries bring a burst of fruity flavor, while almond extract adds a hint of sweetness to this special occasion smoothie.

Fourth of July Berry Blast:

Ingredients:

- 1/2 cup blueberries
- 1/2 cup raspberries
- 1/2 banana
- 1 cup coconut water

Instructions:

Blend until red, white, and blue perfection is achieved.

Benefits This patriotic smoothie is rich in antioxidants and low in sugar, making it a festive and healthy choice.

New Year's Eve Sparkler:

Ingredients:

- 1/2 cup pomegranate seeds
- 1/2 cup blackberries
- 1 tablespoon lime juice
- 1 cup sparkling water

Instructions:

Blend pomegranate seeds, blackberries, and lime juice, then mix with sparkling water.

Benefits This effervescent drink adds a touch of glamour to your New Year's celebration.

Valentine's Day Raspberry Romance:

Ingredients:

- 1/2 cup raspberries
- 1/2 cup strawberries
- 1/2 teaspoon vanilla extract
- 1 cup almond milk

Instructions:

Blend until smooth and romantic.

Benefits This smoothie combines the sweetness of berries with a hint of vanilla, creating a delightful treat for Valentine's Day.

Easter Bunny Carrot Cake:

Ingredients:

- 1/2 cup carrots, shredded
- 1/2 banana
- 1/2 teaspoon cinnamon
- 1 cup unsweetened almond milk

Instructions:

Blend until carroty goodness is achieved.

Benefits This smoothie captures the essence of carrot cake with added fiber and vitamins from fresh carrots.

Halloween Pumpkin Spice Delight:

Ingredients:

- 1/2 cup pumpkin puree
- 1/2 teaspoon pumpkin spice
- 1 tablespoon maple syrup
- 1 cup unsweetened coconut milk

Instructions:

Blend until spooktacular.

Benefits This smoothie provides the beloved flavors of pumpkin spice with minimal added sweetness, making it a festive Halloween treat.

Thanksgiving Harvest Blend

Ingredients:

1/2 cup apple, cored and chopped

1/2 cup pear, peeled and chopped

1/2 teaspoon cinnamon

1 cup unsweetened almond milk

Instructions:

Blend until the flavors of fall come together.

Benefits This smoothie captures the essence of Thanksgiving with a combination of autumn fruits and warm cinnamon.

Conclusion:

Empowering Diabetes Management through Smoothies

In conclusion, the marriage of smoothies and diabetes management represents a dynamic and empowering alliance. Beyond the refreshing sips and vibrant hues, smoothies emerge as a canvas for nutritional ingenuity, offering individuals with diabetes a delectable yet strategic tool to navigate their health journey. The careful selection of ingredients, mindful proportions, and an understanding of the broader impact on overall health elevate smoothies from mere beverages to integral components of a holistic diabetes management plan. As we embark on this exploration of flavors, textures, and nutritional symphony, let the essence of smoothies transcend the glass and become a palatable expression of empowered wellbeing for those with diabetes.